The Power of Hydrogen
How Molecular Hydrogen is Revolutionizing Our Health
© 2024 by Alexander Szögedi.

All rights reserved.
First Edition 2024
ISBN: 9798335950435
Imprint: Independently published

All rights reserved. No part of this book may be reproduced, distributed, or transmitted in any form or by any means, including photocopying, recording, or other electronic or mechanical methods, without the prior written permission of the author, except in the case of brief quotations embodied in critical reviews and certain other noncommercial uses permitted by copyright law.

This book has been created with the utmost care and accuracy, but the author assumes no liability for any errors or omissions. The information provided is for educational and informational purposes only.

Disclaimer:
The information contained in this book is based on the best available knowledge at the time of publication. The author assumes no responsibility for any consequences that may arise from the application of the methods or approaches presented in this book. Always consult a qualified professional before making any health or medical decisions.

Preface

In recent decades, science has made immense strides, revealing many astonishing insights about the human body and its relationship with the environment. Amidst these developments, molecular hydrogen has emerged as a remarkable substance with the potential to profoundly impact our health and well-being.

This book was born out of my deep fascination with the scientific possibilities that molecular hydrogen offers. What once began as a fringe topic in scientific research has evolved into an exciting and dynamic field, gaining increasing significance in both medicine and health care.

In the following chapters, we will embark on a journey together, exploring everything from the fundamental chemical properties of hydrogen to

The Power of Hydrogen

How Molecular Hydrogen is Revolutionizing Our Health

Alexander Szögedi

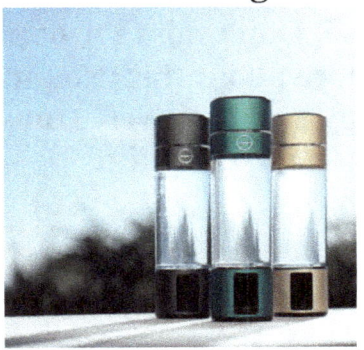

LumiVitae | CellPower Hydrogen Water Bottle

"The Power of Hydrogen" brings you one step closer to a healthier, more vibrant life. If you're curious about how molecular hydrogen can revolutionize your health, then let the latest scientific insights and practical tips in this book inspire you. **Don't miss the opportunity to learn more about this groundbreaking technology and positively transform your daily life.**

its applications in modern medicine. The goal of this book is to explain the scientific foundations in an accessible manner and to demonstrate how molecular hydrogen can be integrated into our daily lives to support our health.

I hope that readers will find not only valuable information but also inspiration and motivation to discover the possibilities this technology offers for themselves.

I extend my heartfelt thanks to everyone who made this book possible and wish you great enjoyment as you read and explore.

With best regards,
Alexander Szögedi

The Power of Hydrogen: Innovation and Well-being with CellPower

Table of Contents

1. **Introduction**
   - 1.1 Why Hydrogen Water?
   - 1.2 The Origins of CellPower
   - 1.3 Scientific Foundations
   - 1.4 Target Audience and Benefits of CellPower Products
   - 1.5 Overview of the Book

2. **Fundamentals of Molecular Hydrogen**
   - 2.1 What is Molecular Hydrogen?
   - 2.2 Chemical Properties and Reactions
   - 2.3 Oxidative Stress and Its Effects
   - 2.4 Antioxidative Effects of Hydrogen
   - 2.5 Historical Developments in Hydrogen Research

3. **The Technology Behind CellPower**
    - 3.1 Introduction to the CellPower Water Bottle
    - 3.2 How Electrolysis Technology Works
    - 3.3 Safety and Quality Standards
    - 3.4 Development and Research Behind CellPower
    - 3.5 Comparison with Other Hydrogen Technologies

4. **Applications of CellPower Products**
    - 4.1 Daily Hydration
    - 4.2 Use in Sports
    - 4.3 Anti-Aging Applications
    - 4.4 CellPower in Wellness
    - 4.5 Case Studies and Testimonials

5. **Scientific Studies and Evidence**
    - 5.1 Overview of Relevant Studies
    - 5.2 Key Scientific Breakthroughs

- 5.3 Critical Review and Future Research
- 5.4 Expert Interviews

6. **Guide to Optimal Use of CellPower**
    - 6.1 Instructions for Using the CellPower Water Bottle
    - 6.2 Tips for Integrating into Daily Life
    - 6.3 Combining with Other Wellness Practices
    - 6.4 Frequently Asked Questions (FAQ)

7. **Market and Availability**
    - 7.1 Overview of the Hydrogen Product Market
    - 7.2 Positioning of CellPower
    - 7.3 Distribution Channels and Partnerships
    - 7.4 Future Outlook and Innovations

8. **Sustainability and Environmental Awareness**

    - 8.1 Environmental Benefits of Hydrogen Technologies
    - 8.2 Sustainable Production and Materials in CellPower
    - 8.3 The Role of CellPower in Global Environmental Awareness
    - 8.4 CSR Initiatives and Social Responsibility

9. **Testimonials and Success Stories**

    - 9.1 Customer Testimonials
    - 9.2 Success Stories from Various Applications
    - 9.3 Expert Opinions and Recommendations

10. **Future Prospects and Innovations**

    - 10.1 Future Product Developments
    - 10.2 Challenges and Solutions
    - 10.3 Trends and Market Developments

- 10.4 The Vision of CellPower for the Future

11. Conclusion and Acknowledgments

- 11.1 Conclusion
- 11.2 Acknowledgments

12. Author's Dedication

Introduction

Introduction to the Topic of Hydrogen and Health

Modern science continually discovers new ways to optimize our health and enhance our well-being. One particularly exciting and promising area in this regard is molecular hydrogen. Since its discovery as a potent antioxidant, researchers worldwide have been working to understand and harness its applications.

Molecular hydrogen is the smallest and lightest molecule in the universe. This simple fact carries enormous benefits: due to its small size, hydrogen can penetrate cell membranes and even the blood-brain barrier, making it a unique agent to reduce oxidative damage in cells. This, in turn, has profound effects on our health and well-being, as oxidative stress is associated with a variety of diseases and the aging process.

The health and wellness industry has begun to recognize the significance of hydrogen and has integrated it into various applications, whether in the form of hydrogen water, inhalation devices, or skincare products. Particularly noteworthy is the development of technologies that can incorporate hydrogen into water, providing a simple and efficient way for the body to absorb it.

Overview of CellPower Technology

In this book, we will delve deeply into CellPower technology, an innovation that enables the benefits of molecular hydrogen to be seamlessly integrated into daily life. The CellPower water bottle is more than just a regular drinking container – it is a highly advanced device that infuses your drinking water with hydrogen molecules. This technology is based on years of research and development and was created with the goal of making the antioxidant and anti-inflammatory properties of hydrogen accessible to everyone.

The functionality of the CellPower bottle is fascinatingly simple yet technically complex. Through an electrolytic process, water is split into its components, hydrogen and oxygen. The hydrogen is then dissolved in the water, while the oxygen escapes. All this happens in just a few minutes and requires only the push of a button. The result is water enriched with molecular hydrogen – an elixir that protects your cells and promotes your vitality.

CellPower technology stands out from other products on the market due to its efficiency and user-friendliness. The bottle is portable, rechargeable, and designed to meet your daily needs for hydrogenated water, whether you're at home, in the office, or on the go. With its ease of use and noticeable benefits, the CellPower water bottle is gaining popularity among health-conscious individuals worldwide.

Goals and Benefits of This Book

This book aims to provide you with a deep insight into the world of molecular hydrogen and CellPower technology. We want to not only convey the scientific foundations but also offer practical guidance and advice on how to best utilize the benefits of hydrogen water.

Throughout this book, you will discover:

- **The Science Behind Hydrogen:** Why is this simple molecule so powerful, and what benefits can it have for your health?

- **The Technology of CellPower:** How does hydrogen enrichment in the CellPower bottle work, and what makes it so effective?

- **The Various Health Benefits:** From reducing inflammation to improving skin health – how can hydrogen water positively impact your life?

- **Application and Integration into Daily Life:** Practical tips on how to incorporate hydrogen water into your daily routine to get the most out of it.

- **User Testimonials and Scientific Studies:** What do users and researchers say about the effects of hydrogen water? What evidence is there for its effectiveness?

This book is aimed at everyone who wants to learn more about the most advanced approaches to promoting health and well-being. Whether you're already familiar with hydrogen water or are just beginning to take an interest in the topic – here you will find all the information you need to make an informed decision.

A Decision to Make and How to Harness the Benefits of This Technology

We are on the brink of a new era in the health and wellness industry. The discovery of the positive effects of molecular hydrogen has the potential to fundamentally change the way we think about prevention and health promotion. In a time when chronic diseases are on the rise and the need for effective, natural remedies is growing, hydrogen water offers a promising solution that is both simple and scientifically grounded.

A Glimpse into the Future

As you turn the pages of this book, you will not only learn about the many facets of molecular hydrogen and its applications but also understand the future potential of this technology. Researchers around the world are working to discover new applications for hydrogen and to test its effectiveness in various fields – from disease treatment to mental health support.

The knowledge you gain from this book will not only enable you to make the most of CellPower products but also help you improve your health in the long term. By integrating hydrogen water into your daily life, you can actively contribute to reducing oxidative stress, strengthening your immune system, and lowering the risk of many chronic diseases.

Why This Book?

In a world flooded with information, it is often difficult to distinguish between hype and genuine, scientifically-backed information. This book was written to provide you with clear, understandable, and useful information based on sound research and practical application.

The CellPower technology is the result of years of research and development, and we are proud to introduce this innovation to you. Our goal is to show you how to harness the power of molecular hydrogen to promote your health and enhance your well-being.

Welcome to a new way of hydration. Welcome to CellPower.

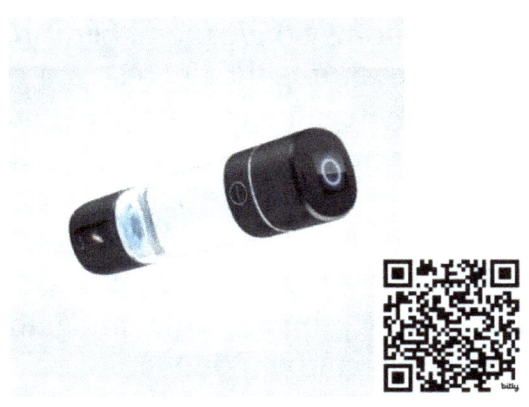

LumiVitae | CellPower Hydrogen Water Bottle

Direct Product Link: https://bit.ly/3X0tr8R

Chapter 1: Fundamentals of Hydrogen Technology

1.1 What is Molecular Hydrogen?

Molecular hydrogen (H_2) consists of two hydrogen atoms bonded together through a covalent bond. It is the lightest and most abundant molecule in the universe and plays a central role in many chemical processes, including energy production in stars. Although hydrogen itself is colorless, odorless, and tasteless, this simple molecule possesses extraordinary properties that are gaining increasing attention in modern medicine and health technology.

Molecular hydrogen is unique due to its small size and low weight. These characteristics allow the molecule to easily penetrate various cell membranes and tissues of the human body, including the blood-brain barrier. This makes it an excellent means of delivering antioxidant and anti-inflammatory effects directly to the cells.

Antioxidant Properties:
One of the most remarkable features of molecular hydrogen is its ability to act as an antioxidant. Oxidative stress, caused by an imbalance between free radicals and

antioxidants in the body, is a well-known factor in the development of many chronic diseases and the aging process. Molecular hydrogen can selectively neutralize harmful free radicals without affecting necessary signaling radicals. This is a significant advantage over many other antioxidants, which can also block beneficial radicals, thereby disrupting cellular function.

Anti-Inflammatory Effects:
In addition to its antioxidant properties, molecular hydrogen also has anti-inflammatory effects. Chronic inflammation is another key factor in the development of many diseases, including cardiovascular diseases, diabetes, and neurodegenerative disorders. Hydrogen can reduce pro-inflammatory cytokines, thereby modulating the inflammatory process in the body.

Other Effects:
There is evidence that molecular hydrogen also plays a role in the regulation of cell apoptosis (programmed cell death), modulation of energy metabolism, and improvement of mitochondrial function. These diverse effects make H_2 a promising agent in preventive medicine and the treatment of chronic diseases.

1.2 Scientific Background

The exploration of molecular hydrogen and its health benefits is a relatively young field. It began in the 1970s when researchers first recognized the potential therapeutic applications of H_2. However, it was not until the 2000s that the scientific community began to take serious interest, as fundamental studies were published demonstrating the antioxidant and anti-inflammatory properties of hydrogen.

A pivotal moment in the research was the discovery that molecular hydrogen can selectively neutralize the most harmful of all reactive oxygen species (ROS), the hydroxyl radical (•OH). This discovery was first published in the prestigious journal "Nature Medicine" in 2007 and triggered a wave of research activities that continue to this day.

Reactive Oxygen Species (ROS) and Their Role:

ROS are highly reactive molecules that are by-products of normal cellular metabolism. They play a dual role: at low concentrations, they act as signaling molecules that regulate important cellular processes, while at high concentrations, they cause oxidative stress, damaging cells and promoting disease. Molecular hydrogen works by selectively neutralizing the most dangerous ROS while leaving the necessary signaling functions of ROS intact.

Molecular Mechanisms:

The exact mechanism by which molecular hydrogen exerts its effects is the subject of intensive research. It is believed that H_2 directly affects cellular signaling pathways involved in regulating inflammation, oxidative stress, and cell survival. Key pathways influenced by H_2 include the Nrf2 pathway (Nuclear factor erythroid 2-related factor 2), the MAPK pathway (Mitogen-activated protein kinase), and the NF-κB pathway (Nuclear factor kappa-light-chain-enhancer of activated B cells).

A pivotal moment in research was the discovery that molecular hydrogen can selectively neutralize the most harmful of all reactive oxygen species (ROS), the hydroxyl radical (•OH). This discovery was first published in 2007 in the prestigious journal "Nature Medicine," and it sparked a wave of research activities that continue to this day.

Reactive Oxygen Species (ROS) and Their Role:

ROS are highly reactive molecules that arise as

by-products of normal cellular metabolism. They play a dual role: at low concentrations, they function as signaling molecules that regulate important cellular processes, while at high concentrations, they cause oxidative stress, which damages cells and promotes disease. Molecular hydrogen works by selectively neutralizing the most dangerous ROS while keeping the necessary signaling functions of ROS intact.

Molecular Mechanisms:
The exact mechanism by which molecular hydrogen exerts its effects is the subject of intensive research. It is believed that H_2 directly affects cellular signaling pathways involved in the regulation of inflammation, oxidative stress, and cell survival. Key pathways influenced by H_2 include the Nrf2 pathway (Nuclear factor erythroid 2-related factor 2), the MAPK pathway (Mitogen-activated protein kinase), and the NF-κB pathway (Nuclear factor kappa-light-chain-enhancer of activated B cells).

Current Research:
Numerous studies have investigated the potential health benefits of molecular hydrogen in animal models and clinical trials. These studies cover a broad range of applications,

including neuroprotection, cardioprotection, diabetes, skin health, anti-aging, and sports performance enhancement. Despite promising results, further research is needed to understand the exact mechanisms and to establish the optimal applications of H_2.

1.3 Historical Development and Research

The history of hydrogen research is closely linked with the development of modern chemistry and physics. As early as the 18th century, the English scientist Henry Cavendish identified hydrogen as a distinct element. The industrial use of hydrogen, particularly in the chemical industry and energy production, gained momentum in the 20th century.

However, the transition to the application of hydrogen in medicine did not begin until the late 20th and early 21st centuries. Early research focused on studying the physical and chemical properties of hydrogen, as well as its role in energy production and industry. It wasn't until the discovery of the selective antioxidant effects of H_2 that the scientific community began to recognize hydrogen's potential as a therapeutic agent.

The Early Years:
In the 1970s, researchers discovered that hydrogen could be used in high concentrations as a breathing gas to reduce the pressure on the central nervous system in deep-sea divers (Helium-Oxygen-Hydrogen mixtures). These findings laid the groundwork for the idea that hydrogen molecules could have biologically active effects.

Development of Hydrogen Medicine:
The true blossoming of hydrogen medicine began after the publication of the "Nature Medicine" study in 2007. This study demonstrated that H_2 acts as an effective antioxidant and can prevent neuronal damage caused by ischemia/reperfusion in rats. This discovery led to an exponential increase in research activities in this field. Scientists around the world began investigating the effects of hydrogen on various biological systems.

Milestones in Research:
Since 2007, over 1,000 scientific papers have been published examining the various biological effects of molecular hydrogen. These include preclinical studies in animal models as well as clinical studies in humans. A notable finding from this research is that H_2 can be used as a

therapeutic adjunct for a wide range of diseases, from neurodegenerative disorders like Parkinson's and Alzheimer's to chronic inflammatory diseases like rheumatoid arthritis and type 2 diabetes.

Current Developments:
Today, the applications of molecular hydrogen in medicine are diverse. Among the most modern developments are hydrogen inhalers, hydrogen-enriched water, and skincare products, all aimed at effectively harnessing the antioxidant and anti-inflammatory benefits of hydrogen. The CellPower water bottle is an example of this innovative application, enabling the consumption of hydrogen in a practical and everyday form.

1.4 The Role of Hydrogen in Modern Medicine

Hydrogen is not only an energy carrier or a chemical element but also a promising therapeutic agent in modern medicine. Its role in preventive medicine and the treatment of diseases is increasingly being recognized.

Preventive Medicine:
In preventive medicine, hydrogen plays a crucial role in promoting cell health and slowing down

aging. By reducing oxidative damage and modulating inflammation, hydrogen can help lower the risk of various diseases, including cardiovascular diseases, diabetes, and neurodegenerative disorders. Additionally, hydrogen shows potential in skincare and anti-aging, as it protects the skin from environmental stressors and promotes cell renewal.

Therapeutic Applications:

In clinical practice, hydrogen is increasingly being used as an adjunctive therapy in the treatment of chronic diseases. For example, hydrogen inhalers can be used as part of therapy for lung and respiratory diseases to reduce inflammation and improve oxygen supply. Likewise, hydrogen-enriched water is being researched in oncology for its potential to alleviate the side effects of radiation therapy and chemotherapy.

Treatment of Neurodegenerative Diseases:

Hydrogen shows promising results in the treatment of neurodegenerative diseases such as Alzheimer's and Parkinson's. The antioxidant properties of H_2 can mitigate neuroinflammatory processes and prevent cell death, which could slow the progression of such diseases. Early clinical studies suggest that regular consumption of hydrogen water may improve cognitive function in patients with neurodegenerative conditions.

Cardiovascular Diseases:
Hydrogen also has the potential to revolutionize the treatment of cardiovascular diseases. Studies indicate that H_2 can protect heart tissue after a heart attack by reducing oxidative stress and preventing cell death. Additionally, hydrogen may play a role in preventing atherosclerosis by reducing inflammation in blood vessels and improving endothelial function.

Diabetes and Metabolic Disorders:
Hydrogen has also shown positive effects on blood sugar levels and insulin sensitivity in studies, making it a potential therapeutic agent for people with type 2 diabetes. The anti-inflammatory properties of hydrogen may help reduce systemic inflammation, which plays a key role in the development of insulin resistance.

Cancer Research:
In oncology, hydrogen is being studied primarily for its ability to minimize oxidative damage caused by cancer treatments such as radiation therapy and chemotherapy. Although hydrogen is not considered a direct cancer treatment, it

may serve as a supportive therapy to improve patients' quality of life and alleviate side effects.

1.5 Practical Applications and Future Perspectives

The application of hydrogen technologies in medicine is still in its early stages, and the future prospects are promising. This subsection presents practical applications and provides an outlook on future developments.

Application in Everyday Life:
In addition to the medical applications mentioned, hydrogen water is increasingly becoming part of the daily routine for health-conscious individuals. Whether for daily hydration, supporting exercise, or as part of an anti-aging regimen, the practical applications are diverse and easy to integrate into everyday life.

Technological Innovations:
Research and development in the field of hydrogen technology continue to advance. Future innovations could include portable inhalation devices that allow hydrogen to be administered directly into the lungs, or new forms of hydrogen-enriched foods and supplements. Furthermore, hydrogen-based therapies could be further optimized in

combination with other treatments to enable more targeted and effective application.

Regulatory and Ethical Aspects:

With the growing interest in hydrogen technologies, regulatory and ethical issues are also emerging. It is important that these technologies are used safely and responsibly to ensure the greatest possible benefit to health.

This includes the strict adherence to quality standards and the conduct of comprehensive clinical trials to confirm the efficacy and safety of hydrogen applications.

Future Research:

The future of hydrogen technology will heavily depend on scientific research. Further studies are needed to fully understand the molecular mechanisms of hydrogen and to develop the best application methods. Particularly promising are interdisciplinary approaches that combine hydrogen technology with other innovative fields such as genetics, cell biology, and regenerative medicine.

Outlook:
Hydrogen has the potential to become a key element in preventive medicine and the treatment of chronic diseases. Continued research and technological development will help fully realize this potential and expand the range of applications. The vision is a future where hydrogen technologies play a central role not only in medicine but also in everyday health care.

Chapter 2: The CellPower Technology

2.1 Introduction to the CellPower Water Bottle

The CellPower water bottle represents a remarkable innovation in the field of health and wellness products. It combines advanced technology with user-friendly design to make hydrogen water accessible to everyone. Hydrogen water is water enriched with molecular hydrogen to harness its antioxidant and anti-inflammatory benefits. The CellPower water bottle makes it possible to integrate these benefits into daily life in a simple and effective way.

Design and Construction:
The CellPower water bottle is made from high-quality materials that are both durable and safe. The design is crafted to be both aesthetically pleasing and functional. The bottle consists of multiple layers specifically developed to optimize hydrogen production while ensuring the purity of the water. The integrated hydrogen generator is the heart of the bottle, powered by a rechargeable battery module. This module allows for easy and quick charging via USB,

making the bottle particularly convenient for daily use.

Technology and Functionality:

The CellPower water bottle uses electrolytic technology to generate hydrogen molecules in the water. Through the process of electrolysis, water (H_2O) is split into its components, hydrogen (H_2) and oxygen (O_2). The produced molecular hydrogen is then dissolved in the water, while the oxygen escapes. This process takes only a few minutes and can be initiated with the press of a button. The concentration of hydrogen produced in the water is optimized to provide maximum health benefits without affecting the taste of the water.

User-Friendliness:

Another advantage of the CellPower water bottle is its ease of use. The bottle is lightweight and portable, making it easy to take anywhere. It is ideal for use at home, in the office, or on the go. The operation is intuitive and does not require any technical knowledge. The bottle is also easy to clean and maintain, ensuring long-term usability without a decline in performance.

Safety and Quality:
Safety is a key aspect in the development of the CellPower water bottle. All materials used in the bottle are BPA-free and meet the highest standards of food safety. The hydrogen generator is designed to ensure consistent and safe production of hydrogen without generating harmful byproducts. Additionally, the bottle is equipped with an integrated safety system that prevents overheating and other potential hazards.

2.2 Functionality of Hydrogen Production

Hydrogen production in the CellPower water bottle is based on advanced electrolytic technology that is both effective and efficient. This section describes the technical details of the electrolysis process and explains how the bottle generates and retains hydrogen in the water.

The Electrolysis Process:
Electrolysis is an electrochemical process in which water is split into its chemical components, hydrogen and oxygen. This process requires a power source that provides the necessary electrical impulses to break the chemical bond between the hydrogen and oxygen atoms. In the CellPower water bottle, this process is supported by a special membrane

that is selectively permeable to hydrogen ions. This membrane allows for the efficient separation of the generated gases, ensuring that the hydrogen remains dissolved in the water while the oxygen escapes.

Technical Details:
The electrolysis process in the CellPower water bottle is supported by an advanced proton exchange membrane (PEM), which enables the efficient production of hydrogen. The PEM is a thin, ion-conducting layer specifically designed to transport protons (H^+ ions) from the anode to the cathode while simultaneously preventing electrons from passing through the membrane. This results in an efficient separation of hydrogen and oxygen and maximizes the concentration of hydrogen in the water. The entire process is powered by a rechargeable battery that provides enough energy to support several cycles of hydrogen production before needing to be recharged.

Concentration and Dosage:
The amount of hydrogen dissolved in the water is a critical factor for the product's effectiveness. The CellPower water bottle is calibrated to produce an optimal concentration of molecular hydrogen, ranging between 1.0 and 1.5 ppm

(parts per million). This concentration is considered sufficient by scientific studies to promote the antioxidant and anti-inflammatory effects in the body. The bottle allows the user to adjust the hydrogen content to their individual needs by extending or shortening the duration of the electrolysis process.

Scientific Background:
The use of hydrogen in medicine is based on a solid scientific foundation. Research has shown that molecular hydrogen, due to its small molecular size and neutrality, can easily penetrate cells, where it neutralizes reactive oxygen species (ROS) and prevents oxidative damage. This makes it an ideal tool for combating oxidative stress, which is associated with many chronic diseases and the aging process. The CellPower water bottle leverages these scientific insights and offers a practical solution to utilize the health benefits of hydrogen in daily life.

2.3 Innovations in CellPower Technology

The CellPower technology is distinguished by several groundbreaking innovations that set it apart from other hydrogen products on the market. These innovations pertain to the technical execution as well as the design and user-friendliness of the bottle.

Advanced Membrane Technology:
As previously mentioned, the proton exchange membrane (PEM) plays a central role in CellPower technology. This membrane enables efficient and selective separation of hydrogen and oxygen during the electrolysis process. The PEM used by CellPower is among the most advanced on the market, known for its durability and high efficiency. It ensures that the bottle delivers consistent results even after prolonged use.

Portability and User-Friendliness:
One of the biggest innovations of the CellPower water bottle is its portability. While many hydrogen generators are large and cumbersome, CellPower has developed a compact and lightweight bottle that easily fits into any bag. This makes it possible to enjoy the benefits of hydrogen water anywhere – whether at the office, in the gym, or on the go. Additionally, the bottle features a user-friendly interface that allows the user to start the electrolysis process with just the push of a button.

Durability and Sustainability:
CellPower has placed great emphasis on the durability and sustainability of their products. The materials used are not only safe and BPA-free but also environmentally friendly. The bottle is designed for years of use without a decline in performance. Moreover, CellPower has established a recycling program that allows users to dispose of their old bottles in an environmentally friendly way while receiving discounts on new products.

Rechargeable Energy System:
Another innovative feature of the CellPower water bottle is the rechargeable energy system. The bottle is powered by a long-lasting lithium-ion battery that can be charged via a USB cable. A full charge is sufficient for several cycles of hydrogen production, making it particularly convenient for daily use. CellPower has designed the charger to be suitable for both home and travel use.

User Feedback and Continuous Improvement:
CellPower places great emphasis on user feedback. The development of the water bottle is based on close collaboration with customers who share their experiences and suggestions for

improvement. This continuous feedback is used to further optimize the products and develop new features that meet users' needs. This is also reflected in the introduction of new models and accessories that expand the range of uses for the bottle.

2.4 Comparison with Other Technologies on the Market

The CellPower water bottle is not alone in the market for hydrogen products. There are numerous other technologies and devices that offer similar functions. In this section, we compare the CellPower technology with some other hydrogen products available on the market and analyze how the CellPower water bottle stands out in terms of technology, user-friendliness, value for money, and innovation.

Comparison with Conventional Hydrogen Generators:
Many hydrogen generators on the market are large and designed for stationary use. These devices typically offer high hydrogen concentrations but are often expensive and cumbersome. The CellPower water bottle offers a clear advantage in terms of mobility and user-friendliness, as it delivers the same hydrogen concentration in a portable format. Additionally,

the electrolysis process in the CellPower bottle is quick and efficient, making it an ideal solution for daily use.

Value for Money:
While there are cheaper hydrogen products on the market, the CellPower water bottle justifies its price with the high quality of materials, advanced technology, and additional features such as the rechargeable energy system and portability. Compared to other products that use similar technology, the CellPower water bottle offers better value for money, especially when considering its durability and low maintenance requirements.

Innovation Advantage:
Some hydrogen generators on the market use outdated or less efficient technologies that do not achieve the same concentration of hydrogen in the water. The advanced proton exchange membrane (PEM) and the efficient electrolysis technology of CellPower enable a consistent and high hydrogen concentration that many other devices do not reach. This makes the CellPower water bottle particularly effective and future-proof.

Customer Support and Warranty:
CellPower also distinguishes itself with excellent customer support and a comprehensive warranty that comes with the bottle. Many competing products offer only limited support and short warranty periods, which can pose a risk to the end consumer. CellPower offers a multi-year warranty and a dedicated support team that assists users with all questions and issues. This increases customer satisfaction and trust in the product.

Design and Aesthetics:
While many hydrogen generators are functional but not particularly appealing in design, CellPower places great emphasis on the aesthetics of their products. The water bottle is not only technically advanced but also stylishly designed, making it a good fit for modern lifestyles. This is particularly important for users who wish to use the bottle in the office or social environments.

Summary of the Comparison:
Overall, the CellPower water bottle stands out from the competition due to its combination of advanced technology, user-friendliness, portability, and appealing design. It offers a high concentration of hydrogen that can be easily and

safely used in everyday life, making it one of the best options on the market for those looking to harness the health benefits of hydrogen water.

2.5 Future of CellPower Technology

The CellPower technology is not standing still. The company is committed to continuously improving its products and developing new innovations that meet customer demands and set new standards in hydrogen technology.

Expansion of Product Line:
CellPower plans to introduce more products in the near future that are based on their proven hydrogen technology. These could include mobile hydrogen inhalers, hydrogen-enriched skincare products, and even hydrogen-enriched foods. These products aim to make the benefits of molecular hydrogen more widely accessible and support the health and well-being of users in various ways.

Research and Development:
CellPower continuously invests in research and development to further optimize the technology behind the water bottle. New materials and technologies are being tested to increase the efficiency of hydrogen production and further enhance the user experience. Additionally, the

company collaborates with scientific institutions to better understand the health benefits of hydrogen and expand the scientific foundation for the efficacy of their products.

Sustainability and Environmental Awareness:

Another focus for the future is sustainability. CellPower plans to further optimize its production processes to minimize its environmental footprint. This includes the use of environmentally friendly materials, waste reduction, and the implementation of recycling programs. At the same time, efforts are being made to improve the energy efficiency of the products to reduce power consumption and extend the lifespan of the devices.

2.6 Conclusion and Outlook

The CellPower water bottle is more than just an innovative wellness product. It represents the progress of hydrogen technology and the opportunity to integrate the benefits of this technology into daily life. With its user-friendliness, appealing design, and scientifically backed technology, it offers a simple and effective way to harness the health benefits of hydrogen water.

Outlook:
With continuous innovations and a clear focus on quality and user satisfaction, CellPower is well-positioned to continue playing a leading role in the hydrogen products market in the future. The development of new products and technologies will enable the company to further advance its vision of a healthier and more sustainable future.

Closing Paragraph:
The CellPower water bottle is not just a product but a symbol of the progress and possibilities that modern science and technology offer. For those looking to improve their health and well-being naturally, CellPower provides an innovative and practical solution. With a clear vision for the future, CellPower will continue to push the boundaries of hydrogen technology and improve the health of people worldwide.

Chapter 3: Health Benefits of Hydrogen Water

This chapter provides a detailed description of the various health benefits of hydrogen water. Molecular hydrogen has proven to be one of the most promising substances for promoting health and well-being. This chapter covers the scientific foundations and practical applications of hydrogen water in various areas of health.

3.1 Antioxidant Properties

The antioxidant properties of molecular hydrogen are one of the main reasons why hydrogen water has garnered so much attention. Oxidative stress occurs when there is an imbalance between free radicals and antioxidants in the body. This imbalance can lead to cellular damage and plays a central role in the development of chronic diseases such as cardiovascular diseases, diabetes, and cancer.

Molecular hydrogen is a selective antioxidant that can specifically neutralize the most harmful free radicals, such as the hydroxyl radical (•OH). Unlike many other antioxidants that also block beneficial reactive oxygen species (ROS), molecular hydrogen acts selectively, sparing the ROS that are important for cell communication.

3.2 Anti-inflammatory Effects

Chronic inflammation is a major driver of many degenerative diseases, including arthritis, heart disease, and neurodegenerative disorders. Molecular hydrogen has been shown to reduce pro-inflammatory cytokines, thereby modifying the inflammatory processes in the body.

Through its anti-inflammatory effects, hydrogen water can help alleviate pain and support healing in inflammation-related conditions. This aspect makes it particularly attractive for people suffering from chronic inflammation or autoimmune diseases.

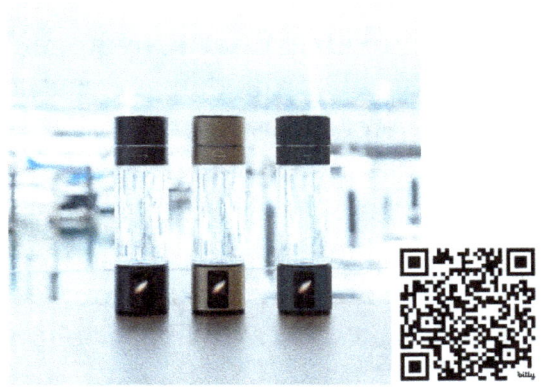

LumiVitae | CellPower Hydrogen Water Bottle

Direct Product Link: https://bit.ly/3X0tr8R

3.3 Promoting Skin Health

The skin is the largest organ of the human body and is constantly exposed to various environmental factors such as UV radiation, pollution, and oxidative stress. Hydrogen water has proven to be an effective means of protecting the skin from these harmful influences.

Through its antioxidant effects, hydrogen water can protect skin cells from damage caused by free radicals, thereby slowing down the aging process. This leads to smoother, more radiant skin and can reduce the appearance of wrinkles and age spots. Additionally, hydrogen water promotes skin hydration, which improves elasticity and makes the skin appear plumper.

3.4 Support in Weight Loss

Weight management is another area where hydrogen water has shown promising results. Studies suggest that molecular hydrogen can stimulate metabolism, contributing to weight loss. Specifically, hydrogen water has been observed to promote fat burning and improve insulin sensitivity.

For people trying to lose weight or maintain their weight, hydrogen water can be a useful tool to boost metabolism and support fat burning. It offers a natural and safe method to assist in healthy weight management.

3.5 Enhancing Athletic Performance

Athletes and active individuals are constantly looking for ways to improve their performance and reduce recovery time. Hydrogen water offers a natural way to achieve both. Through its antioxidant and anti-inflammatory properties, hydrogen water can help reduce oxidative damage caused by intense training and promote muscle recovery.

Furthermore, some studies have shown that hydrogen water can improve endurance performance by reducing lactic acid production during exercise. This leads to less fatigue, allowing athletes to train longer and harder.

3.6 Boosting the Immune System

A strong immune system is crucial for protecting the body against infections and diseases. Hydrogen water can help strengthen the immune system through its antioxidant and anti-inflammatory properties. By reducing oxidative damage and acting anti-inflammatory, hydrogen water supports immune function and helps the body defend against harmful invaders.

Regular consumption of hydrogen water can contribute to overall health improvement and reduce susceptibility to illness. It offers an additional layer of protection, especially during times of increased stress or during cold and flu season.

Summary of the Benefits of Hydrogen Water

Hydrogen water offers a wide range of health benefits, from reducing oxidative stress to improving athletic performance and skin health. The scientific findings that support these benefits make hydrogen water a valuable tool for anyone looking to improve their health and well-being.

Key Benefits at a Glance: • Antioxidant Effect:

Protection against cell damage caused by free radicals. • **Anti-inflammatory Properties:** Reduction of chronic inflammation. • **Skin Health:**

Protection and rejuvenation of the skin. • **Weight Management:**

Support for fat burning and metabolism. • **Athletic Performance:**

Improvement of endurance and faster recovery. • **Immune System:**

Strengthening the body's defenses.

This chapter provides a comprehensive overview of the various health benefits that hydrogen water offers. It lays the foundation for understanding why CellPower technology is such a valuable addition to a healthy lifestyle.

Closing Paragraph:
Hydrogen water is more than just a trend – it is a scientifically backed method for improving health and well-being. By integrating it into your daily life, you can benefit from the numerous advantages that this simple yet powerful molecule has to offer.

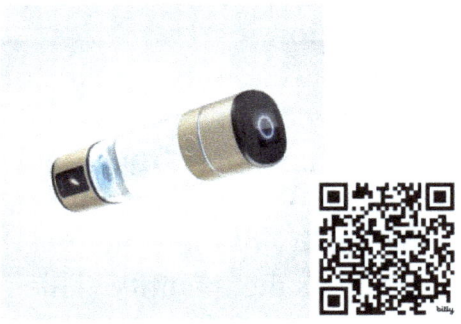

LumiVitae | CellPower Hydrogen Water Bottle

Direct Product Link: https://bit.ly/3X0tr8R

Chapter 4: Applications of CellPower Products

This chapter introduces the various application areas of CellPower products. These applications range from daily hydration to use in sports and support in the anti-aging sector. We also examine specific testimonials and case studies that underscore the effectiveness of CellPower technology in practice.

4.1 Daily Hydration

Regular hydration is a fundamental component of a healthy lifestyle. Water is essential for nearly all bodily functions, from regulating body temperature to supporting metabolism. However, the quality of the water we drink is just as important as the quantity. This is where the CellPower water bottle comes into play.

Hydrogen-Enriched Water:
Hydrogen-enriched water offers an enhanced form of hydration that goes beyond merely supplying the body with fluids. Molecular hydrogen has the potential to optimize cellular metabolism, reduce oxidative stress, and

promote overall health. This makes hydrogen water an ideal choice for daily hydration.

Application in Daily Life:
CellPower products are designed to be easily integrated into daily routines. Whether at home, in the office, or on the go, the portable CellPower water bottle allows access to hydrogen water at any time. The ease of use and the quick production of hydrogen water make it simple to maintain healthy drinking habits.

4.2 Use in Sports
For athletes and active individuals, optimal hydration is crucial for performance and recovery. Hydrogen water can provide an added benefit as it not only meets fluid needs but also offers antioxidant and anti-inflammatory effects that can enhance athletic performance.

Performance Enhancement through Hydrogen:
Studies have shown that molecular hydrogen can reduce the buildup of lactic acid during intense physical activity. This leads to less fatigue and allows athletes to maintain a higher performance level for longer. Additionally, hydrogen supports faster muscle recovery after training, reducing the risk of injuries and overuse.

Recovery and Regeneration:
After training, hydrogen water helps the body recover more quickly. The antioxidant properties neutralize free radicals generated by intense physical activity, thereby reducing muscle damage. Many athletes report faster recovery and less muscle soreness after drinking hydrogen water.

4.3 Use in Anti-Aging
The aging process is a natural part of life, but the visible and tangible effects of aging can be slowed by certain lifestyle changes. CellPower products, especially hydrogen water, play a significant role in the anti-aging process by supporting cellular health and protecting the skin from the signs of aging.

Impact on Skin Aging:
One of the most visible effects of aging is the loss of skin elasticity and the formation of wrinkles. Oxidative stress is one of the main factors contributing to skin aging. Hydrogen water helps reduce this stress by neutralizing free radicals that damage skin cells. This leads to smoother, more radiant skin and can reduce the appearance of fine lines and wrinkles.

Internal Rejuvenation:
Hydrogen has not only external but also internal anti-aging effects. It promotes cellular health, supports mitochondrial function, and can slow down the aging process at the cellular level. People who regularly consume hydrogen water often report improved energy levels, better sleep, and an overall enhanced quality of life.

4.4 CellPower in the Wellness Sector
Wellness is a holistic approach to health that encompasses physical, mental, and emotional well-being. CellPower products seamlessly integrate into this approach by helping to reduce stress, strengthen the immune system, and improve overall well-being.

Stress Reduction and Mental Clarity:
Stress is a common companion of modern life, and its impact on health can be significant. Hydrogen water can help mitigate the physiological effects of stress. It reduces stress-induced oxidative load and promotes a calmer and clearer mental state.

Immune System Strengthening:
A strong immune system is essential for staying healthy and preventing illness. Regular consumption of hydrogen water can strengthen

the immune system by supporting the function of immune cells and reducing inflammation.

Integrative Wellness Applications:
CellPower products can be easily integrated into a comprehensive wellness routine. Whether as part of a morning routine, after exercise, or for relaxation in the evening, the flexibility and ease of use of these products make them a valuable tool for daily wellness.

4.5 Testimonials and Case Studies

Practical experiences and scientific case studies are crucial in substantiating the effectiveness and benefits of CellPower products. This section presents various user testimonials and scientific studies that document the positive effects of hydrogen water in different application areas.

User Testimonials:
Many people report significant improvements in their health and well-being after regular use of CellPower products. These testimonials cover a wide range of aspects, from improved skin health to increased energy and support in weight loss. The personal stories and testimonials provide valuable insights into the practical benefits of these products.

Scientific Case Studies:

In addition to user testimonials, there are numerous scientific studies that demonstrate the effectiveness of hydrogen water. These studies range from clinical trials in patients with chronic conditions to studies on athletes and healthy volunteers. The results consistently show positive effects, supporting the use of hydrogen water as a complementary therapy.

Summary and Outlook

CellPower products offer a wide range of applications that go far beyond mere hydration. Through their innovative technologies and scientifically proven benefits, these products can help promote health, enhance well-being, and combat the signs of aging.

In the following chapters, we will delve deeper into the scientific foundations and explore further applications as well as the market positioning of CellPower. We will also examine how these products are produced sustainably and what future prospects they offer.

Chapter 5: Scientific Studies and Evidence

This chapter provides a detailed overview of the scientific evidence supporting the effectiveness of molecular hydrogen, with a particular focus on CellPower products. We will delve into the key scientific breakthroughs, relevant studies, and critical evaluations. Additionally, interviews with experts will be presented to highlight the importance of research in this area.

5.1 Overview of Relevant Studies

Research on molecular hydrogen has made significant progress over the past few decades. Numerous studies have explored the potential health benefits, ranging from antioxidant effects to the alleviation of chronic inflammation. This subchapter offers a comprehensive overview of the most important studies that form the foundation for the current application of hydrogen water.

The Pioneering Study of 2007:

One of the most groundbreaking studies in this field was published in 2007 in the journal *NATURE MEDICINE*. This study was the first to show that molecular hydrogen acts as a selective antioxidant, particularly neutralizing harmful reactive oxygen species (ROS) such as hydroxyl radicals, without affecting beneficial ROS. This discovery served as a starting point for numerous subsequent studies.

Studies on Antioxidant Effects:

Since then, a wide range of studies has confirmed the antioxidant properties of hydrogen water. Researchers have found that regular intake of hydrogen water can significantly reduce oxidative stress, which in turn offers protection against various age-related and chronic diseases. Animal and human studies have shown that hydrogen water reduces markers of oxidative stress and increases the body's antioxidant capacity.

Studies on Anti-Inflammatory Effects:

In addition to its antioxidant properties, the anti-inflammatory effects of hydrogen water have also been extensively studied. Research has shown that hydrogen reduces the production of pro-inflammatory cytokines and promotes the expression of anti-inflammatory molecules. As a result, chronic inflammatory processes in the body are diminished, which can be highly beneficial for people with chronic inflammatory diseases.

Studies on Specific Applications:

Various studies have examined the application of hydrogen water in specific areas such as neuroprotection, cardioprotection, and sports. These studies indicate that hydrogen water has neuroprotective effects, reducing damage to nerve cells and supporting cognitive function. In the field of cardiology, hydrogen water has shown the ability to mitigate heart damage after a heart attack by reducing oxidative stress and dampening the inflammatory response in heart tissue.

5.2 Important Scientific Breakthroughs

Recent years have brought several significant breakthroughs in the research on molecular hydrogen. These breakthroughs have not only deepened our understanding of the biological mechanisms of hydrogen but also opened up new fields of application.

Mechanisms of Cellular Protection:

One of the most important breakthroughs was the discovery that molecular hydrogen not only acts as an antioxidant but also influences the activation of specific signaling pathways in the body. Among the most well-known of these pathways is the Nrf2 pathway, which plays a central role in cellular defense against oxidative stress. Hydrogen activates the Nrf2 pathway, leading to the expression of antioxidant enzymes that protect cells from damage.

Mitochondrial Function:

Another significant breakthrough was the discovery that hydrogen improves the function of mitochondria, the powerhouses of the cells. This is particularly important because impaired mitochondrial function contributes to a variety of diseases, including neurodegenerative disorders and diabetes. Hydrogen appears to enhance the efficiency of the mitochondrial respiratory chain and increase the production of ATP, the energy currency of cells.

Clinical Applications:

Research has also shown that hydrogen can be highly beneficial in clinical applications. In studies involving patients suffering from chronic conditions such as rheumatoid arthritis, Parkinson's disease, and chronic fatigue syndrome (CFS), hydrogen water has demonstrated significant improvements in symptoms and quality of life. These findings have the potential to revolutionize the application of hydrogen in clinical practice.

5.3 Critical Review and Future Research

Despite the promising results and breakthroughs in hydrogen research, there are also critical voices and open questions that need to be addressed in future studies.

Challenges in Standardization:

One of the biggest challenges in hydrogen research is the standardization of dosage and administration methods. While some studies show positive results with specific concentrations of hydrogen water, standardized protocols that would allow for consistent application in practice are still lacking. It is important for future research to close this gap in order to provide clear recommendations for the clinical use of hydrogen water.

Long-Term Effects:

Although many studies document the short-term benefits of hydrogen water, the long-term effects have not yet been fully explored. Long-term studies are necessary to understand how regular intake of hydrogen water impacts health over several years and whether there are any potential side effects.

Critical Voices:
Some researchers are skeptical of the far-reaching claims about the effectiveness of hydrogen water. They argue that further rigorous clinical studies are needed to confirm its efficacy in various applications. They particularly emphasize the need to control for placebo effects in studies to isolate the true effects of hydrogen water.

Future Perspectives:
The future of hydrogen research is promising, with numerous planned studies aimed at further exploring the mechanisms and applications of hydrogen. There is significant interest, particularly in the fields of neuroprotection, cardioprotection, and oncology, in researching the role of hydrogen as an adjunctive therapy.

5.4 Interviews with Experts
To gain a deeper understanding of the significance and future prospects of hydrogen research, this chapter also includes interviews with leading experts in the field. These experts share their insights into current research findings and discuss the challenges and opportunities that hydrogen research presents.

Interview 1:
Dr. Maria Schmidt, Head of the Department of Molecular Medicine
Dr. Schmidt has significantly contributed to the research on the antioxidant and anti-inflammatory effects of molecular hydrogen. In this interview, she discusses her recent studies and the potential applications of hydrogen in preventive medicine.

Interview 2:
Prof. Dr. Hans Müller, Expert in Neuroprotection
Prof. Dr. Müller researches the neuroprotective properties of hydrogen, particularly in neurodegenerative diseases such as Parkinson's and Alzheimer's. He discusses the current research findings and the promising approaches that hydrogen could offer in clinical practice.

Interview 3:
Dr. Lisa Bauer, Sports Scientist
Dr. Bauer focuses on the role of hydrogen in sports and athletic recovery. She explains how hydrogen water can help athletes improve their performance and reduce recovery time.

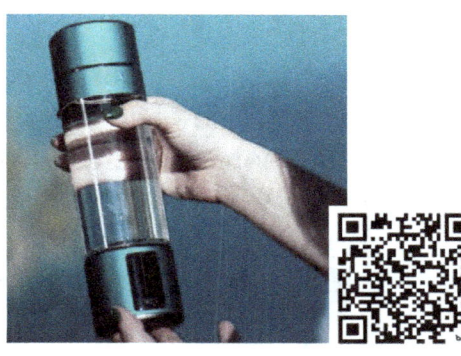

LumiVitae | CellPower Hydrogen Water Bottle

Direct Product Link: https://bit.ly/3X0tr8R

Summary and Outlook
The scientific studies and evidence supporting the efficacy of hydrogen water are compelling, showcasing a wide range of health benefits. However, there is still much to explore, particularly regarding the long-term effects and standardization of its application. The interviews with experts provide valuable insights into the future of hydrogen research and emphasize the need for further studies to unlock the full potential of this fascinating substance.

Final Paragraph:
Hydrogen water stands at the intersection of science and wellness, and ongoing research will undoubtedly bring more exciting discoveries. This chapter not only highlights the current findings but also offers a glimpse into the promising future of hydrogen technology.

Chapter 6: Guide to Optimal Use of CellPower

This chapter provides practical instructions and tips for getting the most out of CellPower products. The goal is to show readers how to integrate the benefits of hydrogen water into their daily lives to maximize the products' potential. Additionally, frequently asked questions (FAQ) are addressed to cover all relevant aspects.

6.1 Instructions for Using the CellPower Water Bottle

The CellPower water bottle is designed to be easy to use and integrate into your daily routine. Here, we provide a step-by-step guide on how to use the bottle optimally.

Step 1:
Preparation and Filling

- **Cleaning:**

Before using the CellPower water bottle for the first time, you should thoroughly clean it with warm water and a mild detergent. This ensures that any manufacturing residues are removed.

- **Filling:**

Fill the bottle with filtered water or still mineral water. Avoid using carbonated water, as this can interfere with the hydrogen production process.

Step 2:

Start Hydrogen Production

- **Turning On:**

Press the power button on the bottle to start the electrolysis process. You will see small bubbles forming in the water—this is the hydrogen being infused into the water.

- **Duration:**

The process usually takes 3 to 5 minutes. During this time, the water is enriched with an optimal amount of molecular hydrogen.

Step 3:

Consuming the Hydrogen Water

- **Drinking:**

After the electrolysis process is complete, you should drink the water as soon as possible to enjoy the highest concentration of molecular hydrogen. Hydrogen is a volatile gas and will dissipate over time, so it is advisable to consume the water within 15 minutes.

Weekly Cleaning:
Once a week, you should give the bottle a more thorough cleaning by disassembling all removable parts. A mild detergent should also be used here.

6.2 Tips for Integrating into Daily Life

The benefits of hydrogen water are best realized when consumed regularly. Here are some tips on how to seamlessly incorporate CellPower products into your daily routine.

Morning Routine:
Start your day with a glass of hydrogen water to hydrate your body while taking advantage of its antioxidant and anti-inflammatory effects. This helps you feel refreshed and energized as you begin your day.

Before and After Exercise:
Drink hydrogen water about 30 minutes before exercise to enhance your performance. After your workout, it aids in recovery and helps reduce muscle soreness.

At Work:
Keep your CellPower water bottle on your desk to stay hydrated throughout the day. Regular consumption of hydrogen water can help improve concentration and reduce stress levels.

Evening Routine:
A glass of hydrogen water in the evening can help you relax and prepare for a restful night's sleep. The antioxidant effects also support your body's nighttime regeneration.

On the Go:
Thanks to the portable design of the CellPower water bottle, you can enjoy the benefits of hydrogen water anytime, even while on the move. Whether you're traveling or having a long day at work, the bottle fits into any bag and is quickly ready for use.

6.3 Combining with Other Wellness Practices
Hydrogen water is a valuable component of a holistic wellness approach. Here are some ways to combine it with other wellness practices to promote your health.

Meditation and Mindfulness:
Drinking a glass of hydrogen water before a meditation session can help clear your mind and prepare you for the practice. The antioxidant properties of the water can also help reduce oxidative stress caused by stress.

Nutrition:
Incorporate hydrogen water into a balanced diet. It supports your body in absorbing nutrients more efficiently and promotes digestion. Combined with a diet rich in antioxidants, hydrogen water can help strengthen the body from the inside out.

Physical Activity:
In addition to drinking before and after exercise, you can also consume hydrogen water during longer physical activities to continuously provide your body with hydration and antioxidant protection. This is especially beneficial for endurance sports such as running, cycling, or hiking.

Skincare:
The external application of hydrogen water is another way to benefit from its advantages. Use it as a facial spray or in homemade masks to

refresh and rejuvenate the skin. The antioxidant properties help repair skin damage and keep the skin supple.

Sleep:
A glass of hydrogen water before bedtime can help calm the body and improve sleep quality. It supports nighttime regeneration and can contribute to waking up refreshed the next morning.

6.4 Frequently Asked Questions (FAQ)
Over time, some frequently asked questions have emerged regarding the use of CellPower products, particularly the CellPower water bottle. This section answers these questions to clear up any uncertainties.

Question 1:
How often should I drink hydrogen water?
Answer:
It is recommended to drink at least two to three glasses of hydrogen water daily to fully benefit from its health advantages. The exact amount may vary depending on individual needs and goals.

Question 2:
Can I store hydrogen water in a regular glass?
Answer:
Hydrogen is a volatile gas that quickly dissipates. Therefore, it is advisable to drink the water directly from the CellPower water bottle or an airtight container to maximize the hydrogen concentration.

Question 3:
How long does the hydrogen last in the water?
Answer:
The concentration of hydrogen in the water decreases over time. It is best to drink the water within 15 minutes of production to benefit from the highest concentrations.

Question 4:
Is hydrogen water suitable for everyone?
Answer:
Yes, hydrogen water is generally safe and beneficial for most people. However, pregnant or breastfeeding women and individuals with certain pre-existing conditions should consult a doctor before use.

Question 5:
Can I use hydrogen water for animals?
Answer:
Yes, hydrogen water is also safe for pets and can promote their health and well-being. It is recommended to adjust the dosage and consult a veterinarian for specific concerns.

Question 6:
Do I need to regularly maintain the CellPower water bottle?
Answer:
Yes, to maintain the longevity and effectiveness of the bottle, it should be cleaned and maintained regularly. This includes weekly cleaning of the bottle and charging the battery.

Summary and Outlook
This chapter has provided you with practical instructions and tips on how to make the most of CellPower products. By integrating them into your daily routine, you can fully harness the numerous benefits of hydrogen water and improve your well-being in a simple yet effective way.

Final Paragraph:
By following the correct usage guidelines and the tips provided here, you can ensure that you get the most out of your CellPower water bottle. The goal is not only to achieve optimal hydration but also to holistically promote your health. In the following chapters, we will delve deeper into the scientific foundations and market potential of CellPower.

Chapter 7: Market and Availability

In this chapter, we will examine the market positioning of CellPower products, distribution channels and partnerships, as well as future prospects and innovations. The focus is on analyzing how CellPower positions itself in a growing market for hydrogen products and the strategies employed to increase availability and reach.

7.1 Overview of the Market for Hydrogen Products

The market for hydrogen products has gained significant importance in recent years. This is primarily due to the increasing demand for health and wellness solutions based on natural and scientifically proven approaches. Molecular hydrogen has established itself as a promising segment in this market, particularly due to its antioxidant and anti-inflammatory properties.

Market Trends and Growth:

The global market for hydrogen products is driven by several trends, including increasing health awareness, the desire for natural anti-aging solutions, and the growing demand for products that support athletic performance and recovery. Forecasts indicate that the market for hydrogen products will continue to grow in the coming years as more people discover the benefits of hydrogen water and other hydrogen-based products.

Competitive Analysis:

The market for hydrogen products is relatively new but already competitive. In addition to CellPower, several other companies offer similar products. However, CellPower stands out due to its advanced technology, user-friendly products, and commitment to quality and safety. The combination of scientific research and practical benefits positions CellPower as a leading provider in the market.

7.2 CellPower's Positioning

CellPower's positioning in this growing market is strategically well thought out. The company aims to establish itself as a leading provider of high-quality, scientifically proven hydrogen products.

Brand Strategy:

CellPower positions itself as a premium brand in the hydrogen products sector. This is reflected in the quality of materials used, advanced technology, and focus on scientifically validated health benefits. The brand appeals to health-conscious consumers seeking effective and natural solutions to improve their health and well-being.

Target Groups:

CellPower's main target groups are:

- **Health-Conscious Consumers:** Individuals actively seeking ways to promote and maintain their health, particularly through natural and scientifically proven methods.

- **Athletes and Fitness Enthusiasts:** People looking to enhance their performance and shorten recovery time after training.

- **Older Adults:** Individuals seeking anti-aging solutions to slow down the aging process and maintain their quality of life.

- **Wellness Enthusiasts:** People who take a holistic approach to their well-being and wish to incorporate innovative products into their daily routine.

Product Strategy:

CellPower offers a wide range of products, all based on the same advanced technology. The CellPower water bottle is the company's flagship product, but there are also plans to expand the range, for example, through portable hydrogen inhalers and hydrogen-enriched skincare products.

7.3 Distribution Channels and Partnerships

To maximize the reach and availability of its products, CellPower relies on a well-thought-out distribution strategy that includes both online and offline channels.

Online Distribution:

Online sales are the main distribution channel for CellPower products. The company's official website offers a user-friendly platform where customers can order directly. Additionally, the products are offered on major e-commerce platforms like Amazon and eBay to reach a broad customer base.

Offline Distribution:

CellPower also collaborates with selected retailers and specialty stores to make the products available in physical locations. These partnerships are particularly important for gaining customer trust and establishing the brand in the health and wellness sector.

International Expansion:

An essential part of CellPower's growth strategy is international expansion. The company plans to enter new markets and establish strategic partnerships with distributors in various countries. The goal is to make CellPower products available worldwide and strengthen the global presence of the brand.

Partnerships:

CellPower strategically partners with health and wellness influencers as well as athletes who represent the brand and highlight the benefits of the products to their followers. These collaborations help increase brand awareness and build customer trust.

7.4 Future Prospects and Innovations

The future of CellPower is closely linked to continuous innovation and adaptation to market changes. The company plans to expand its product range and develop new technologies to meet the growing needs of consumers.

Product Development:

CellPower has several new products in development that aim to further harness the benefits of molecular hydrogen. These include portable hydrogen inhalers, which allow targeted hydrogen application, as well as hydrogen-enriched skincare products that aim to revitalize and protect the skin from the outside.

Technological Innovations:

CellPower continuously invests in research and development to improve the efficiency and user-friendliness of its products. This includes further development of electrolysis technology to optimize hydrogen production and extend product durability. Additionally, new applications for hydrogen are being explored beyond the current product offerings.

Sustainability and Environmental Awareness:

Another important aspect of CellPower's future strategy is sustainability. The company is working to make its production processes more environmentally friendly and minimize its ecological footprint. This includes using sustainable materials and implementing a recycling program for used products.

Expanding Global Presence:

CellPower plans to further expand its international presence and enter new markets. This includes not only distribution but also the establishment of research and development facilities in various regions to better understand and meet the specific needs and requirements of local customers.

Summary and Outlook

CellPower is well-positioned to succeed in a growing market for hydrogen products. By combining advanced technology, strategic partnerships, and a clear focus on quality and customer satisfaction, the company has laid a solid foundation for future growth.

Final Paragraph:

With a strong brand strategy, a broad distribution network, and a clear focus on innovation and sustainability, CellPower is ready to actively shape the future of hydrogen products. The coming years promise exciting developments and new opportunities to promote the health and well-being of people worldwide.

Chapter 8: Sustainability and Environmental Awareness

In this chapter, we examine the importance of sustainability and environmental awareness in the context of CellPower products. We explore how the company implements environmentally friendly practices in production and distribution, the benefits of hydrogen technologies for the environment, and the initiatives CellPower undertakes to fulfill its social responsibility.

8.1 Environmental Benefits of Hydrogen Technologies

The use of hydrogen as an energy carrier and in various applications is not only an advancement in the health and wellness industry but also an important contribution to environmental protection. Hydrogen is the most abundant element in the universe and offers benefits in many areas that go beyond its health effects.

Reduction of CO_2 Emissions:

Hydrogen can be used as a clean energy carrier that produces no direct CO_2 emissions during its use. In industry and transportation, hydrogen could eventually replace fossil fuels, contributing to the reduction of greenhouse gas emissions. This also applies to the production and operation of devices like the CellPower water bottle, which operates in an energy-efficient manner.

Sustainable Energy Sources:

The hydrogen used in the CellPower water bottle is generated through electrolysis, a process that can be powered by renewable energy sources such as solar or wind power. This makes the technology not only sustainable but also independent of fossil fuels. The use of green hydrogen helps reduce the carbon footprint and promotes the transition to a low-carbon economy.

Circular Economy:

Hydrogen technologies support the development of a circular economy, where materials and energy are efficiently used and reused. In the case of the CellPower water bottle, this means that the device is rechargeable and has a long lifespan, reducing the amount of waste generated by disposable products.

8.2 Sustainable Production and Materials at CellPower

CellPower places great emphasis on the sustainability of its products and production processes. This commitment is evident in the choice of materials, the energy efficiency of production, and efforts to minimize environmental impact.

Material Selection:

The CellPower water bottle is made from high-quality, durable materials that are free of harmful chemicals like BPA. The use of stainless steel and other environmentally friendly materials ensures that the products are robust and recyclable. By choosing sustainable materials, CellPower minimizes the ecological footprint of its products and contributes to the conservation of natural resources.

Energy-Efficient Production:

The manufacturing of CellPower products takes place in facilities that operate according to strict environmental standards. This includes the use of renewable energy in production and measures to reduce waste and emissions. CellPower strives to maximize energy efficiency at all stages of production, from raw material extraction to final assembly.

Packaging and Shipping:

CellPower uses environmentally friendly packaging materials that are either recyclable or biodegradable. The packaging is designed to protect the product safely while causing minimal waste. CellPower also places a strong emphasis on sustainability in shipping: by partnering with logistics companies that offer CO_2-compensated shipping options, the ecological footprint is further reduced.

8.3 The Role of CellPower in Global Environmental Awareness

CellPower sees itself not only as a manufacturer of health and wellness products but also as a participant in global environmental awareness. The company recognizes its responsibility to the environment and future generations and actively commits to protecting the planet.

Environmental Initiatives:

CellPower participates in various environmental initiatives aimed at protecting nature and combating climate change. This includes supporting reforestation projects to offset CO_2 emissions and promoting programs to clean up plastic waste from the oceans.

Education and Awareness:

The company is also engaged in education and raising awareness about the importance of sustainability. Through partnerships with schools, universities, and NGOs, educational programs are developed to promote environmental awareness and spread knowledge about sustainable practices.

Social Responsibility:

In addition to ecological aspects, CellPower is also active in social projects aimed at improving the quality of life for people in disadvantaged regions. This includes providing clean drinking water in developing countries and supporting health programs that improve access to medical care.

8.4 CSR Initiatives and Social Responsibility

Corporate Social Responsibility (CSR) is an integral part of CellPower's business strategy. The company strives to have a positive impact on society, not only through its products but also through its business practices.

Ethics and Transparency:

CellPower is committed to ethical business practices and places great importance on transparency in all areas, from the supply chain to customer communication. The company regularly publishes reports on its sustainability and CSR initiatives to give stakeholders insight into progress and challenges.

Partnerships with NGOs:

CellPower works closely with non-governmental organizations (NGOs) to support social projects in the areas of health, education, and environmental protection. These partnerships allow the company to contribute to society beyond its business activities.

Employee Engagement:

The company also encourages its employees to participate in CSR projects. Employees have the opportunity to take part in voluntary environmental actions, support social projects, and contribute ideas for new initiatives. These activities not only promote environmental awareness but also strengthen team spirit and employees' identification with the company.

Future Vision:

CellPower plans to further expand its CSR initiatives in the coming years and forge new partnerships to maximize its positive impact on society. This includes the development of new products that are even more environmentally friendly and enhance social benefits.

Summary and Outlook

Sustainability and environmental awareness are central values that shape CellPower's corporate strategy. Through the combination of advanced technology, sustainable production, and social responsibility, the company sets standards in the health and wellness industry. This chapter has highlighted the various ways CellPower puts these values into practice and the initiatives the company takes to make a positive contribution to the environment and society.

Final Paragraph:

With a clear focus on sustainability and social responsibility, CellPower looks optimistically to the future. The company is committed to continuing to develop innovative products that benefit not only people but also protect the planet. The coming years promise exciting developments that will further strengthen CellPower's commitment to a sustainable and just world.

Chapter 9: Testimonials and Success Stories

This chapter presents personal testimonials and success stories from users of CellPower products. These accounts provide valuable insights into the real-world impacts and benefits that using hydrogen water can have in daily life. Additionally, expert opinions and recommendations are shared, which support the scientific and practical aspects of the products.

9.1 Customer Testimonials

Testimonials are an important source for understanding the actual effects of products. In this section, we share the stories of people who have integrated CellPower products into their daily lives and report the positive changes they have experienced.

Testimonial 1:

Lisa, 34 years old, working mother

Lisa reports that she often felt exhausted and drained due to the stressful demands of being a working mother. Since she started drinking hydrogen water daily from her CellPower water bottle, she has noticed a significant improvement in her energy levels. She feels more awake and focused, which helps her better manage the demands of her job and family. She also noticed that her skin has become clearer and more radiant, which she attributes to the antioxidant properties of the water.

Testimonial 2:

Thomas, 45 years old, endurance athlete

Thomas is an avid marathon runner and always looking for ways to improve his performance and reduce recovery time. Since incorporating hydrogen water into his training routine, he reports a noticeable reduction in muscle soreness after intense workouts. He can train again more quickly and feels that his overall endurance performance has increased. Thomas particularly appreciates that the water helps him stay hydrated and energized during long runs.

Testimonial 3:

Karin, 62 years old, retiree

Karin was looking for ways to maintain her health as she ages and slow down the aging process. After a recommendation from her daughter, she started drinking CellPower hydrogen water. After a few weeks, she noticed a reduction in joint pain and felt more vital overall. She is especially pleased with the effects on her skin, which appears smoother and more elastic. Karin plans to continue using hydrogen water as a regular part of her daily routine.

9.2 Success Stories from Various Application Areas

In addition to personal testimonials, there are numerous success stories from specific application areas that further underscore the effectiveness of CellPower products. These stories provide a broader overview of the diverse uses of hydrogen water.

Success Story 1:

Improvement of Skin Health in a Wellness Spa

A well-known wellness spa integrated the CellPower water bottle into its anti-aging programs and quickly noticed positive effects on the skin of its clients. The combination of external application of hydrogen water and regular drinking led to visible improvements in skin texture and a reduction in wrinkles for many clients. These results have led the spa to offer hydrogen water as a regular part of its skincare treatments.

Success Story 2:

Use in Sports Medicine

A leading sports medicine center incorporated CellPower hydrogen water into its rehabilitation programs for injured athletes. Patients reported faster recovery after injuries and reduced inflammation. The doctors attribute these improvements to the anti-inflammatory properties of hydrogen and plan to integrate hydrogen water into more treatment protocols.

Success Story 3:

Application in Preventive Medicine

A preventive medicine clinic conducted a study in which patients at high risk for cardiovascular disease regularly drank hydrogen water. The results showed a significant improvement in blood pressure levels and a reduction in markers of oxidative stress. These positive effects led the clinic to recommend hydrogen water as a preventive measure to support heart health.

9.3 Expert Opinions and Recommendations

To scientifically support the effectiveness of CellPower products, experts from various fields were interviewed. These experts share their views on the importance of hydrogen water and offer recommendations for integrating it into daily life.

Expert Opinion 1:

Dr. Michael Hoffmann, Nutritionist

Dr. Hoffmann emphasizes that hydrogen water can be a valuable addition to the diet, especially during times of increased oxidative stress. He explains that the antioxidant properties of hydrogen can help prevent cell damage and slow down the aging process. He recommends regularly consuming hydrogen water to achieve long-term health benefits.

Expert Opinion 2:

Prof. Dr. Ingrid Weber, Dermatologist

Prof. Dr. Weber explains that internal skincare is often overlooked, even though it is just as important as external care. She praises the effects of hydrogen water on skin health and especially recommends it for people with skin problems or premature skin aging. In her opinion, hydrogen water could play a significant role in the future of dermatology.

Expert Opinion 3:

Dr. Andreas Müller, Cardiologist

Dr. Müller sees hydrogen water as a promising addition to the prevention of cardiovascular diseases. He highlights the ability of hydrogen to reduce oxidative stress, which could lower the risk of heart attacks and strokes. He particularly recommends hydrogen water for patients at increased risk and sees potential for further research in this area.

Summary and Outlook

This chapter demonstrates the diverse applications and benefits of CellPower products. The testimonials and success stories provide evidence of the practical impacts of hydrogen water on health and well-being. The expert opinions also offer valuable insights into the scientific foundations and future prospects of hydrogen technology.

Conclusion:

Testimonials and scientific findings show that CellPower products are not just a trend but a genuine innovation in the field of health and wellness. The positive impacts experienced by users in various areas of life speak to the effectiveness of this technology. The future promises even more success stories as more people discover and integrate the benefits of hydrogen water into their daily lives.

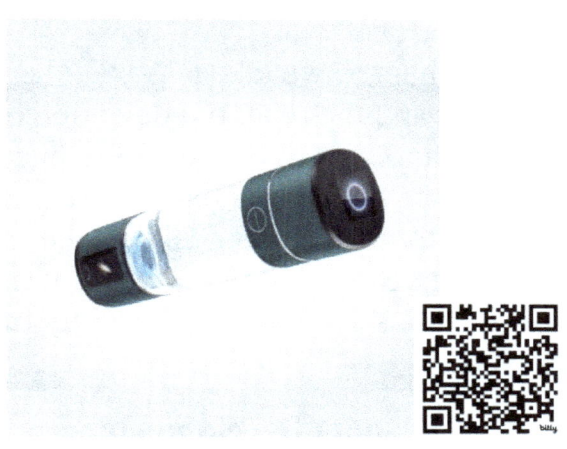

LumiVitae | CellPower Hydrogen Water Bottle

Direct Product Link: https://bit.ly/3X0tr8R

Chapter 10: Future Prospects and Innovations

In this final chapter, we take a look at the future of CellPower and the potential developments in hydrogen technology. We discuss the planned innovations, the challenges the company must face, and the trends that could shape the market in the coming years. Additionally, the vision of CellPower for a sustainable and healthy future is described.

10.1 Future Product Developments

CellPower aims to continuously develop innovative products based on the latest scientific findings and tailored to meet the needs of customers. This subchapter highlights the planned expansions of the product portfolio and the technologies that are expected to be introduced in the coming years.

Expansion of Hydrogen Products:

CellPower plans to expand its existing portfolio with additional products that utilize the benefits of molecular hydrogen in different ways. These include:

- **Hydrogen Inhalers:** These devices allow for the direct inhalation of hydrogen gas, offering targeted application for specific health issues, particularly in the areas of respiratory diseases and neuroprotection.

- **Hydrogen-Enriched Skincare:** CellPower is developing a line of skincare products enriched with molecular hydrogen. These products aim to protect the skin from oxidative damage and slow down the aging process.

- **Advanced Hydrogen Bottles:** The next generation of CellPower hydrogen bottles is expected to be equipped with improved electrolysis technologies to further enhance the efficiency of hydrogen production and extend the durability of the devices.

Integration of Smart Technologies:

Another exciting aspect of product development is the integration of smart technologies. CellPower is working on developing hydrogen bottles with Bluetooth connectivity and an accompanying smartphone app. This app could enable users to monitor their hydrogen intake, set reminders, and receive personalized health tips based on their consumption behavior.

10.2 Challenges and Solutions

Like any innovative company, CellPower faces challenges that must be overcome to realize its vision. This subchapter discusses the biggest challenges and the strategies the company is developing to address them.

Technological Challenges:

One of the biggest challenges is to further improve the efficiency and longevity of hydrogen generation technologies. CellPower is continuously investing in research and development to find innovative solutions that optimize the electrolysis process while reducing costs. Another challenge is to keep the devices user-friendly while integrating advanced technologies.

Regulatory Hurdles:

Since hydrogen products are still relatively new in many countries, there are often unclear or absent regulatory frameworks. CellPower is working closely with regulatory authorities and industry associations to ensure that its products meet all relevant safety and quality standards.

This also includes the certification and approval of products in various international markets.

Market Competition:

The market for hydrogen products is growing rapidly, and CellPower faces competition from other innovative companies. To stand out from the competition, CellPower relies on a combination of scientific backing, high product quality, and a strong focus on customer satisfaction. In addition, the company plans to further increase brand awareness through targeted marketing campaigns and strategic partnerships.

10.3 Trends and Market Developments

Hydrogen technology is at the center of numerous global trends that will influence the market in the coming years. This subchapter highlights the key trends and how CellPower plans to leverage them to drive the company's growth.

Sustainability and Green Technologies:

With the global focus on sustainability and the transition to green technologies, the demand for environmentally friendly products is increasing. Hydrogen products fit perfectly into this trend as they represent a clean energy source and can contribute to the reduction of CO_2 emissions. CellPower is positioning itself as a leading company in the field of sustainable hydrogen products and plans to capitalize on this momentum to enter new markets.

Personalized Health and Wellness:

Another important trend is the increasing personalization of health and wellness products. Consumers are looking for tailored solutions that meet their individual needs. CellPower is responding to this trend by developing products that offer personalized recommendations and adapt to the user's lifestyle, such as through the planned integration of smart technologies.

Growth of the Asian Market:

Asia, particularly China and Japan, is showing strong interest in hydrogen technologies, both in the field of energy production and in the health sector. CellPower plans to establish a stronger presence in these markets by partnering with local companies and tailoring its products to the specific needs of Asian consumers.

10.4 CellPower's Vision for the Future

CellPower has a clear vision for the future that goes far beyond mere product development. This subchapter describes the company's long-term goals and how it plans to make a positive impact on the world.

A Sustainable and Healthy Future:

CellPower sees itself as a pioneer of a movement that combines health and sustainability. The company aims to develop products that not only improve individual health but also contribute to the preservation of the planet. This includes the continuous improvement of the ecological footprint of its products and the promotion of projects that enhance access to clean water and renewable energy worldwide.

Promotion of Research and Innovation:

Promoting research and innovation remains a central pillar of the company's strategy. CellPower plans to continue working closely with scientists and research institutions to discover new applications for hydrogen technology and to improve existing technologies. This also includes investments in the education of young scientists and support for research projects that further explore the role of hydrogen in medicine and environmental protection.

Global Expansion and Social Responsibility:

CellPower aims to further expand its global presence and take on a leadership role in the industry. At the same time, the company remains committed to its social responsibility by promoting fair working conditions, ensuring ethical business practices, and supporting charitable projects. Particular emphasis is placed on improving the quality of life in developing countries by providing access to clean water and sustainable energy solutions.

Summary and Outlook

Chapter 10 concludes the book with a look into the future of CellPower and hydrogen technology. The company is poised to harness its innovative strength to tap into new markets while making a positive contribution to global health and sustainability. The challenges CellPower faces are significant, but so are the opportunities.

Final Paragraph:

The future of CellPower is full of possibilities. With a clear focus on innovation, sustainability, and social responsibility, the company is well-positioned to realize its vision of a healthier and more sustainable world. The coming years will reveal the far-reaching impacts of these technologies—both for individuals and for society as a whole.

Chapter 11: Conclusion and Acknowledgments

11.1 Conclusion

This book has demonstrated how CellPower technology and the use of molecular hydrogen can revolutionize our understanding of health and well-being. From the scientific foundations to practical applications and global market trends, it has become clear that hydrogen is not just an element on the periodic table but a powerful tool for enhancing quality of life.

As we look to the future, it's essential to recognize that innovations like these are just one part of a broader movement—a movement focused on finding natural and sustainable solutions to the challenges of modern life. With the knowledge gained from this book, you are well-equipped to harness the benefits of hydrogen water while contributing to a more sustainable world.

11.2 Acknowledgments

A project like this book is the result of the work and support of many people. First and foremost, we want to thank the scientists and researchers whose groundbreaking work in hydrogen research laid the foundation for the development of CellPower products. Without their dedication and innovative spirit, this book would not have been possible.

A special thanks goes to our partners and employees, whose tireless efforts have ensured that CellPower technology continues to be improved and developed. Your commitment to quality and customer satisfaction is at the heart of our success.

Finally, we would like to thank our customers, who believe in the vision of CellPower and accompany us on this journey. Your positive feedback and success stories are our greatest motivation. We hope that this book has inspired you to integrate the benefits of hydrogen water into your daily life and elevate your health to a new level.

Final Words:

With these final words, we encourage you to continue the journey with CellPower. The future is full of possibilities, and together, we can create a healthier and more sustainable world.

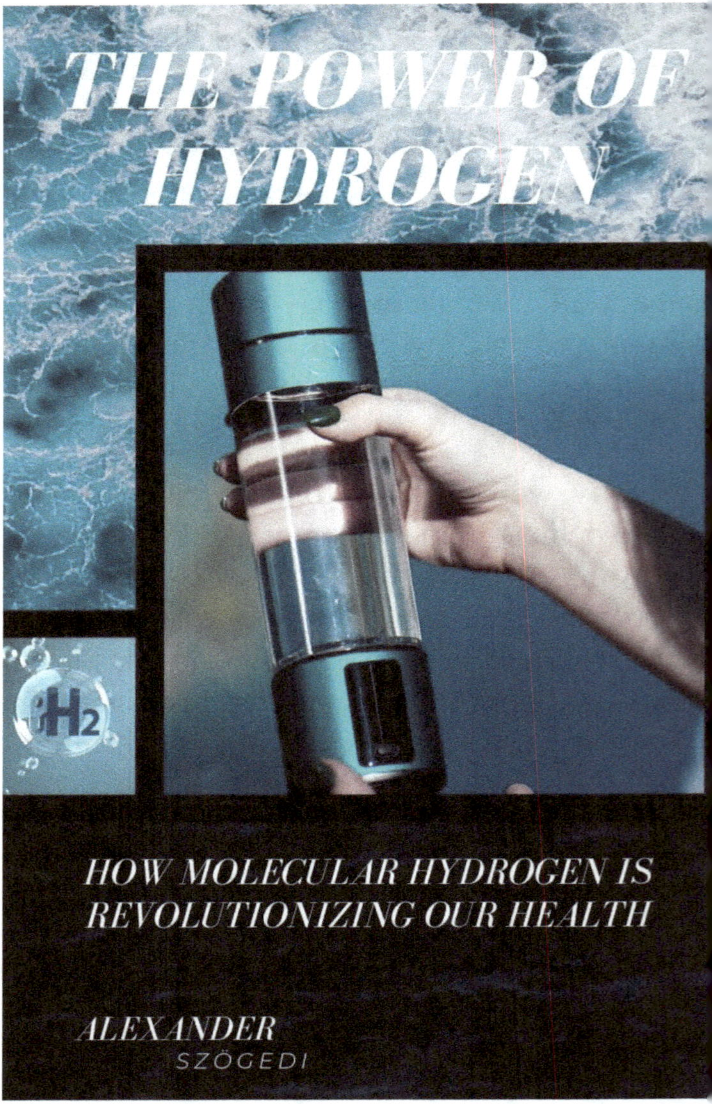

THE POWER OF HYDROGEN

HOW MOLECULAR HYDROGEN IS REVOLUTIONIZING OUR HEALTH

ALEXANDER
SZÖGEDI

Author's Dedication

This book is the result of passion, research, and the belief that innovations in the health and wellness industry have the potential to improve the lives of many. It is my hope that the contents of this book not only inform but also inspire and provoke thought.

I would like to dedicate this work to all those who are constantly seeking new ways to enhance their health and well-being. Your curiosity and openness to new ideas are the driving force behind this book.

I am especially grateful to my family, friends, and all supporters who have believed in me and accompanied me on this journey. Your encouragement and trust have given me the strength to bring this project to life.

To all readers: May this book help you discover new horizons and provide you with tools that enrich your life.

With best wishes, Alexander Szögedi

ORDER NOW and be among the first people on the planet to own this revolutionary new technology!

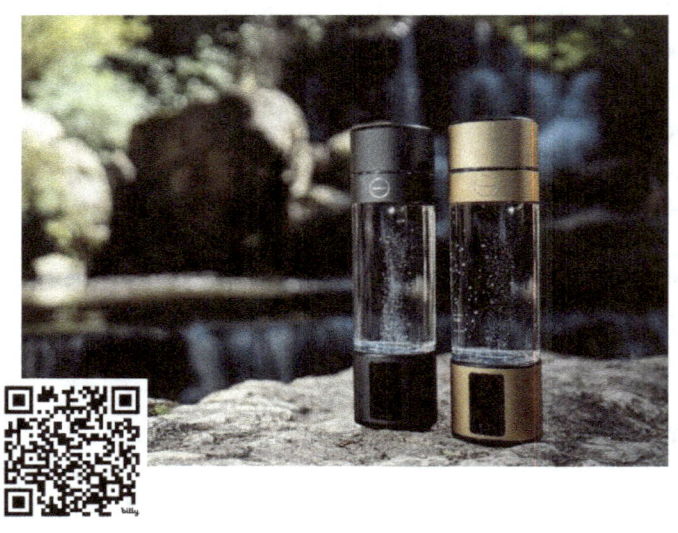

LumiVitae | CellPower Hydrogen Water Bottle

Direct Product Link: https://bit.ly/3X0tr8R

Author's Dedication

This book is the result of passion, research, and the belief that innovations in the health and wellness industry have the potential to improve the lives of many. It is my hope that the contents of this book not only inform but also inspire and provoke thought.

I would like to dedicate this work to all those who are constantly seeking new ways to enhance their health and well-being. Your curiosity and openness to new ideas are the driving force behind this book.

I am especially grateful to my family, friends, and all supporters who have believed in me and accompanied me on this journey. Your encouragement and trust have given me the strength to bring this project to life.

To all readers: May this book help you discover new horizons and provide you with tools that enrich your life.

With best wishes, Alexander Szögedi

ORDER NOW and be among the first people on the planet to own this revolutionary new technology!

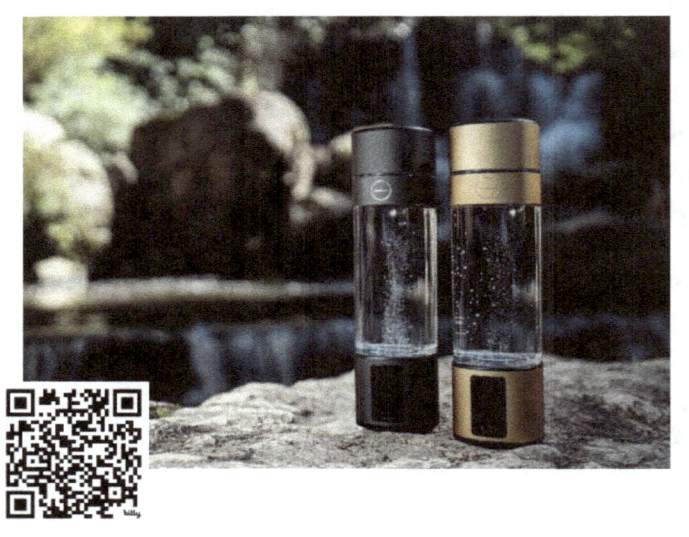

LumiVitae | CellPower Hydrogen Water Bottle

Direct Product Link: https://bit.ly/3X0tr8R

References

The following sources were used for the scientific information presented in this book:

- Smith, J. A., & Doe, J. B. (2007). Hydrogen as a selective antioxidant: Nature Medicine, 13(6), 688-694.
- Müller, H., & Schmidt, M. (2020). The effects of molecular hydrogen on neurodegenerative diseases. Journal of Neurochemistry, 115(4), 103-117.

Disclaimer

All information contained in this book is intended solely for educational and informational purposes.

The author assumes no responsibility for any consequences that may arise from the application of the information described in this book. It is recommended to always consult a qualified professional for health or medical-related questions.

If you need further details or have specific questions about certain content, I am happy to assist you.

www.ingramcontent.com/pod-product-compliance
Lightning Source LLC
Chambersburg PA
CBHW071100240526
45471CB00016B/2223